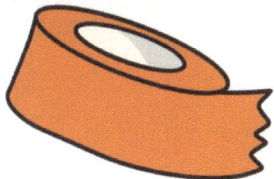
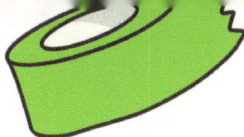

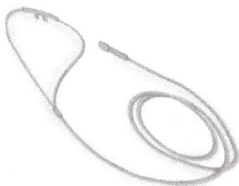
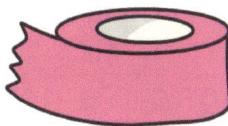
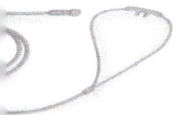
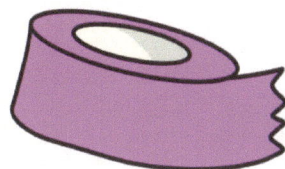
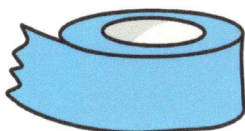
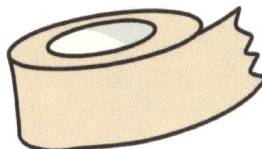
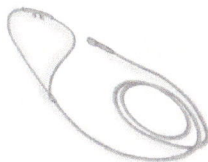
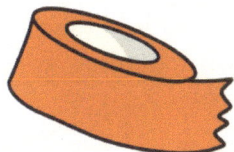
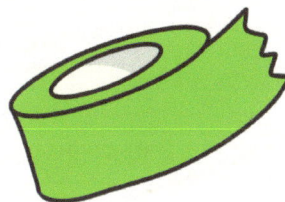
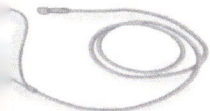
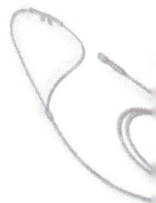
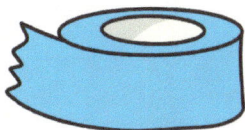
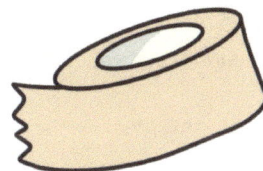
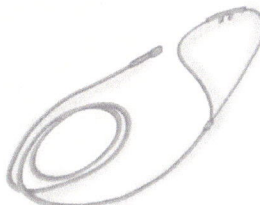
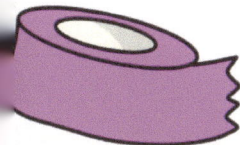
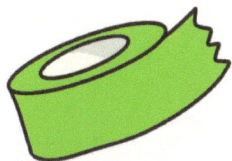
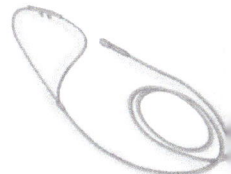
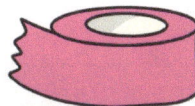

For all the parents going through the oxygen journey.
You are not alone x

My Oxygen Baby

Written and Illustrated by
Lisa McArthur-Collins

First Printing, 2024

Published by Little Wings Publishing
www.littlewingspublishing.com

ABN 31 448 359 874

ISBN 978-0-6486471-2-6 Paperback version
ISBN 978-0-6486471-3-3 Hardcover version
ISBN 978-0-6486471-4-0 eBook version

My Oxygen Baby

Written and Illustrated by

Lisa McArthur-Collins

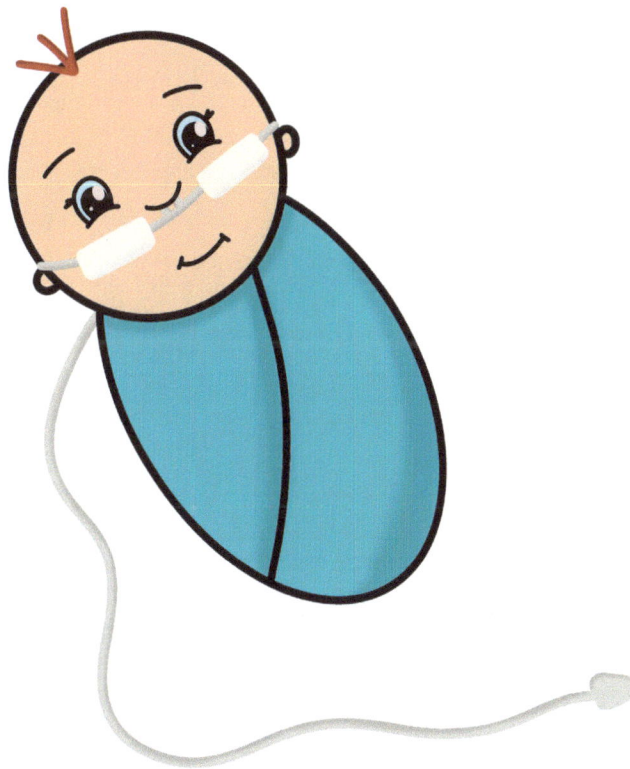

The oximeter beeps all through the night,

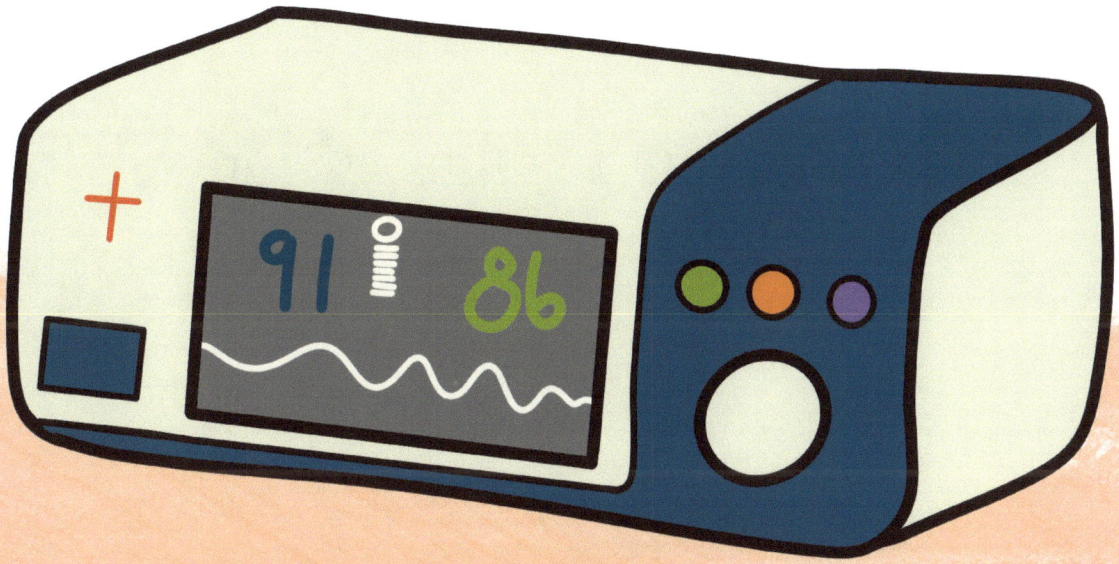

The doctor said you need some help,
so you can learn to breathe just right.

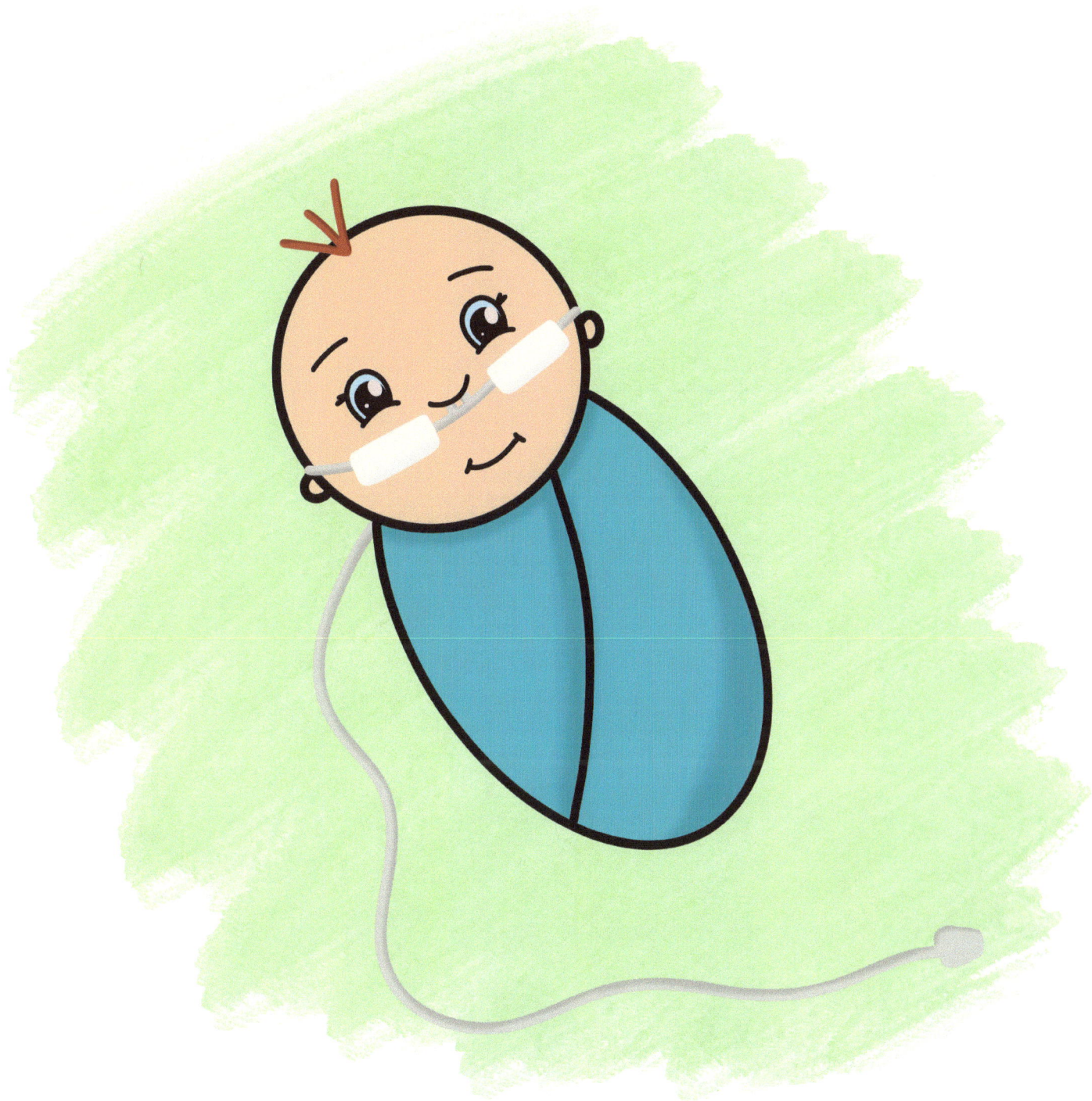

Nasal cannulas, oxygen tubes,
rolls and rolls of coloured tape,

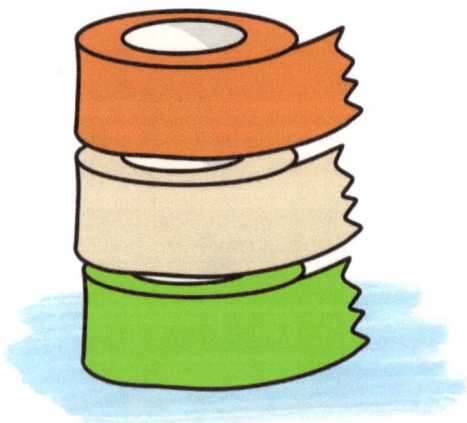

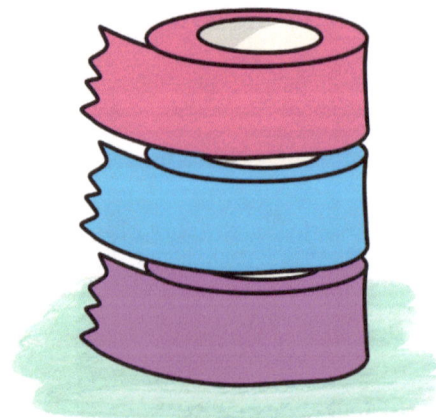

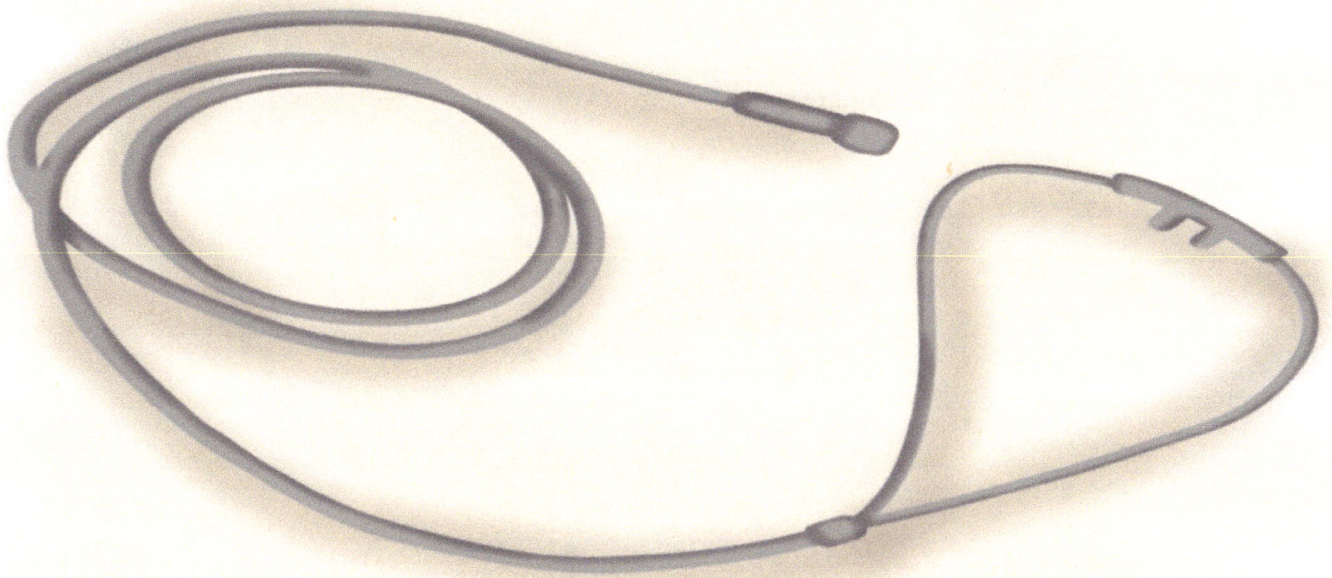

Oxygen cylinders are everywhere,
they are hard to escape.

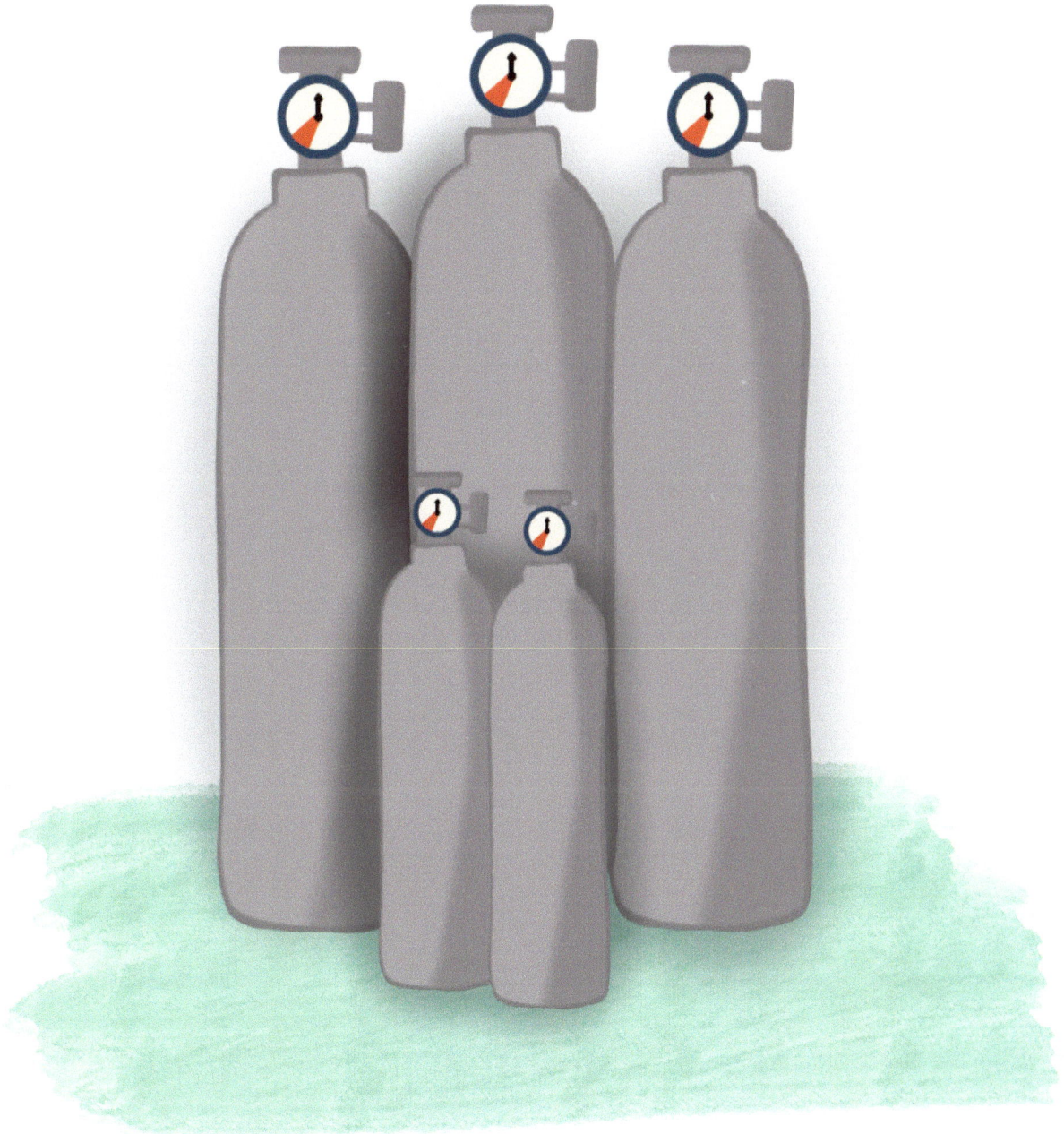

They go with us whenever we leave our home,

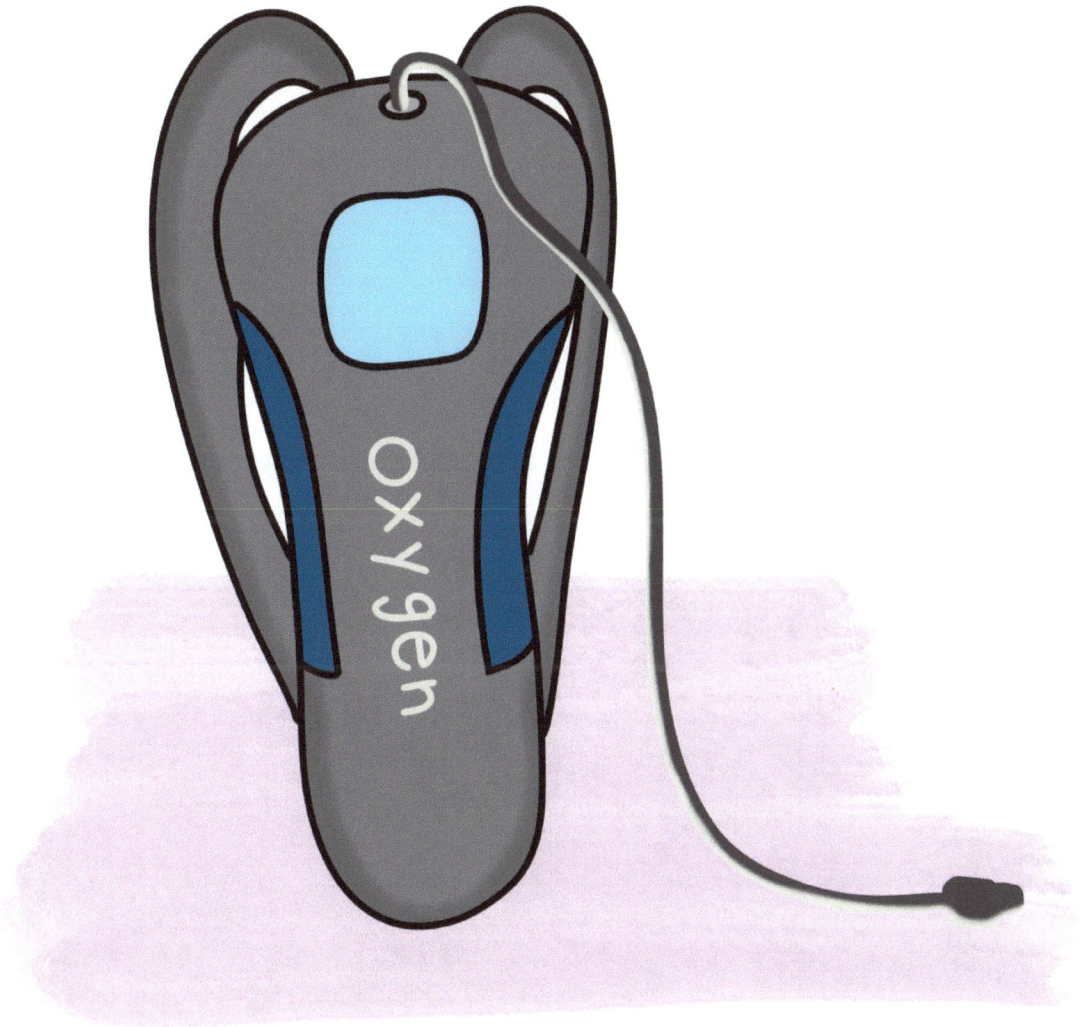

This gives us the freedom to get out and roam.

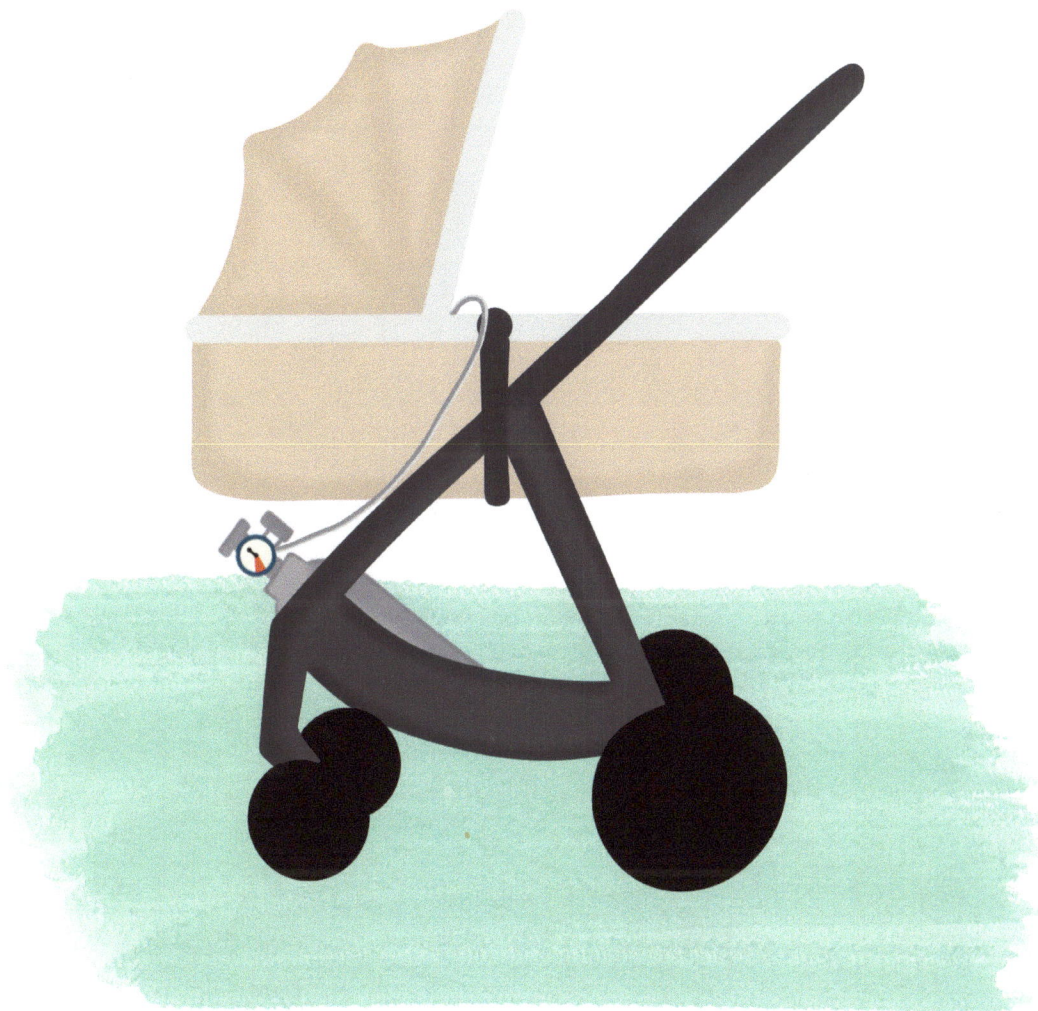

After each sleep study,
we have too long to wait,

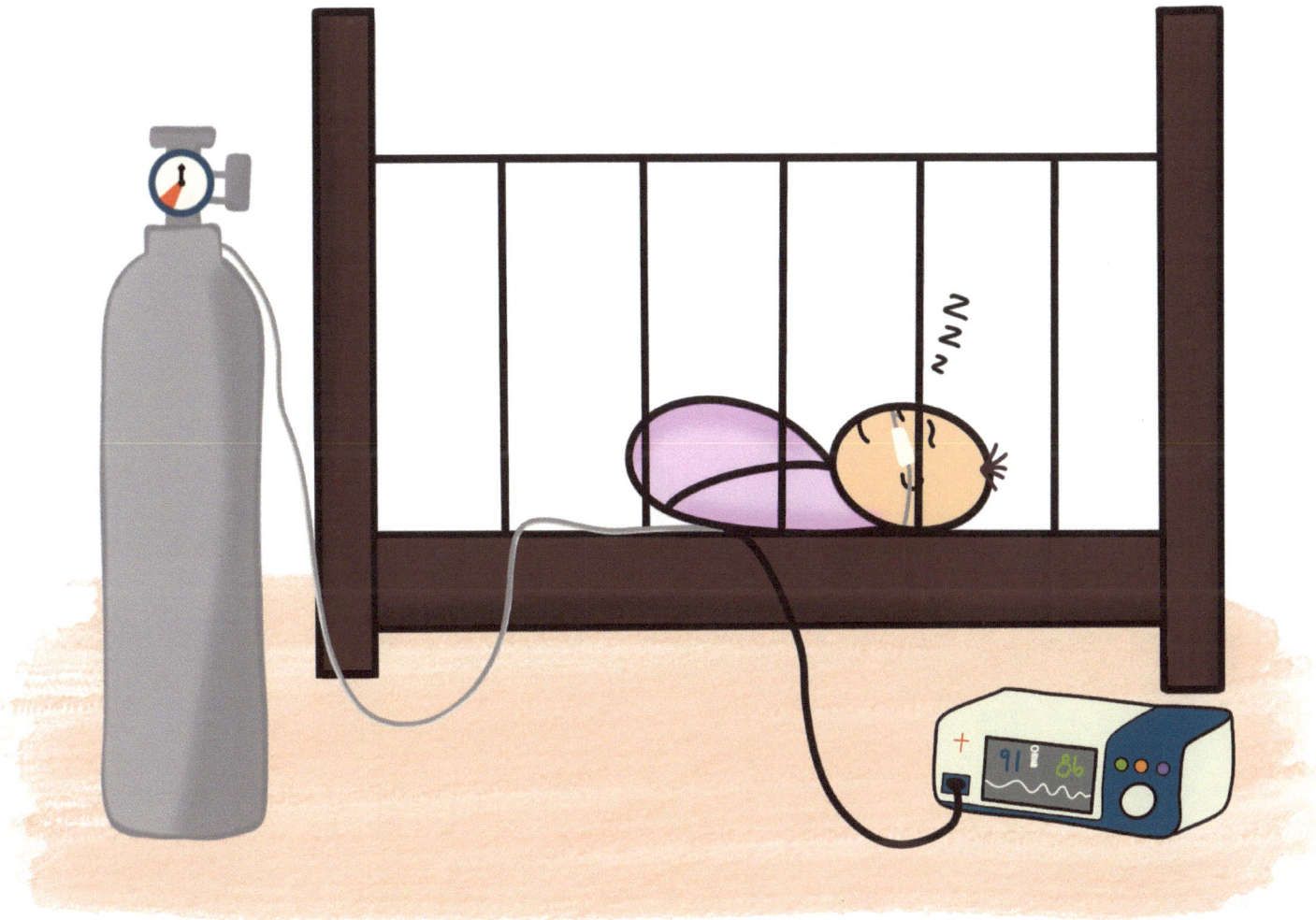

It feels like forever as we pray
and wait for the date.

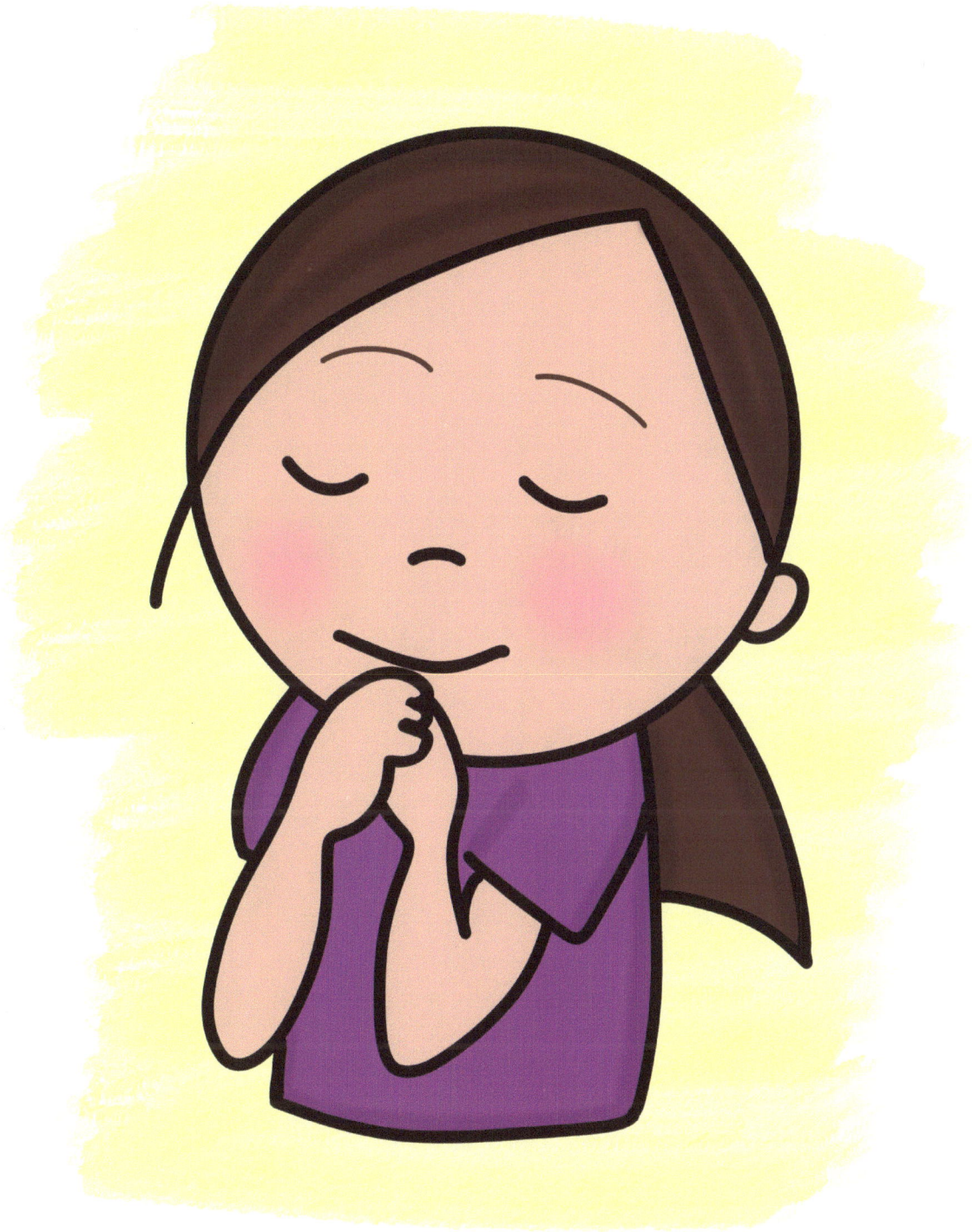

The results mean that you're not yet

ready to breathe alone,

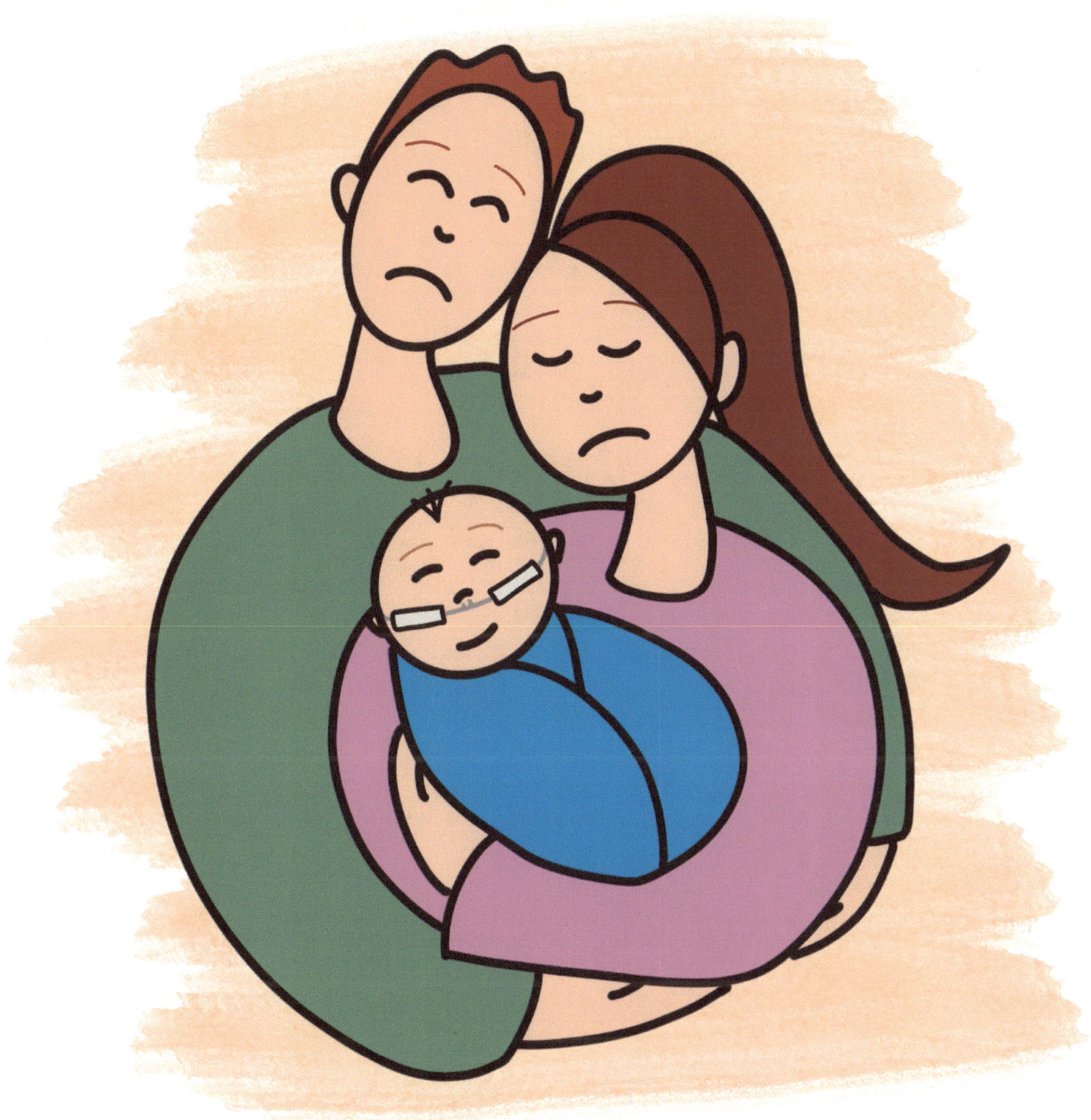

The future feels so unknown.

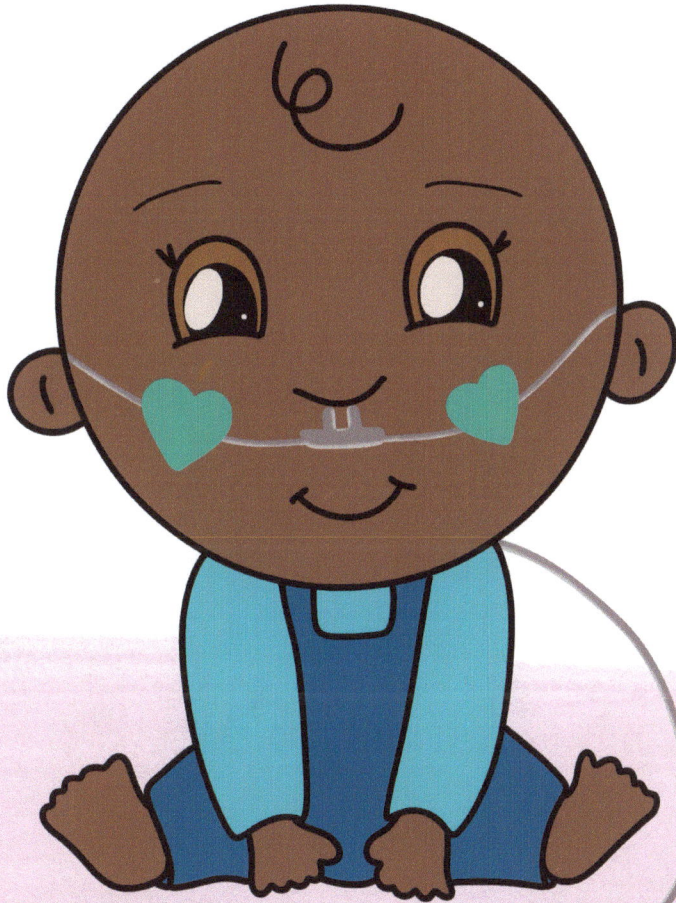

We dream of the day we'll see
your beautiful face,

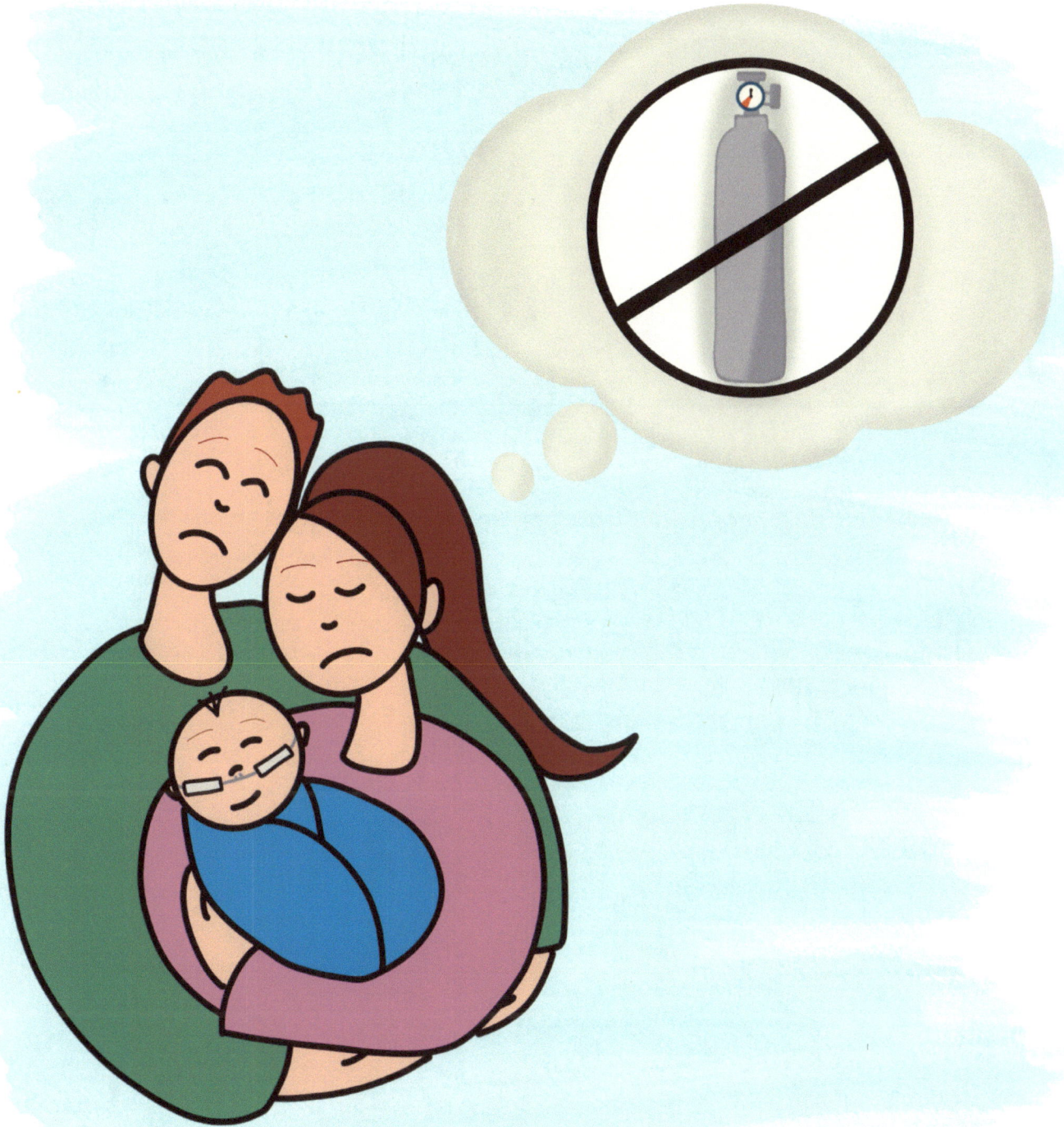

Without these oxygen tubes,
that feel so out of place.

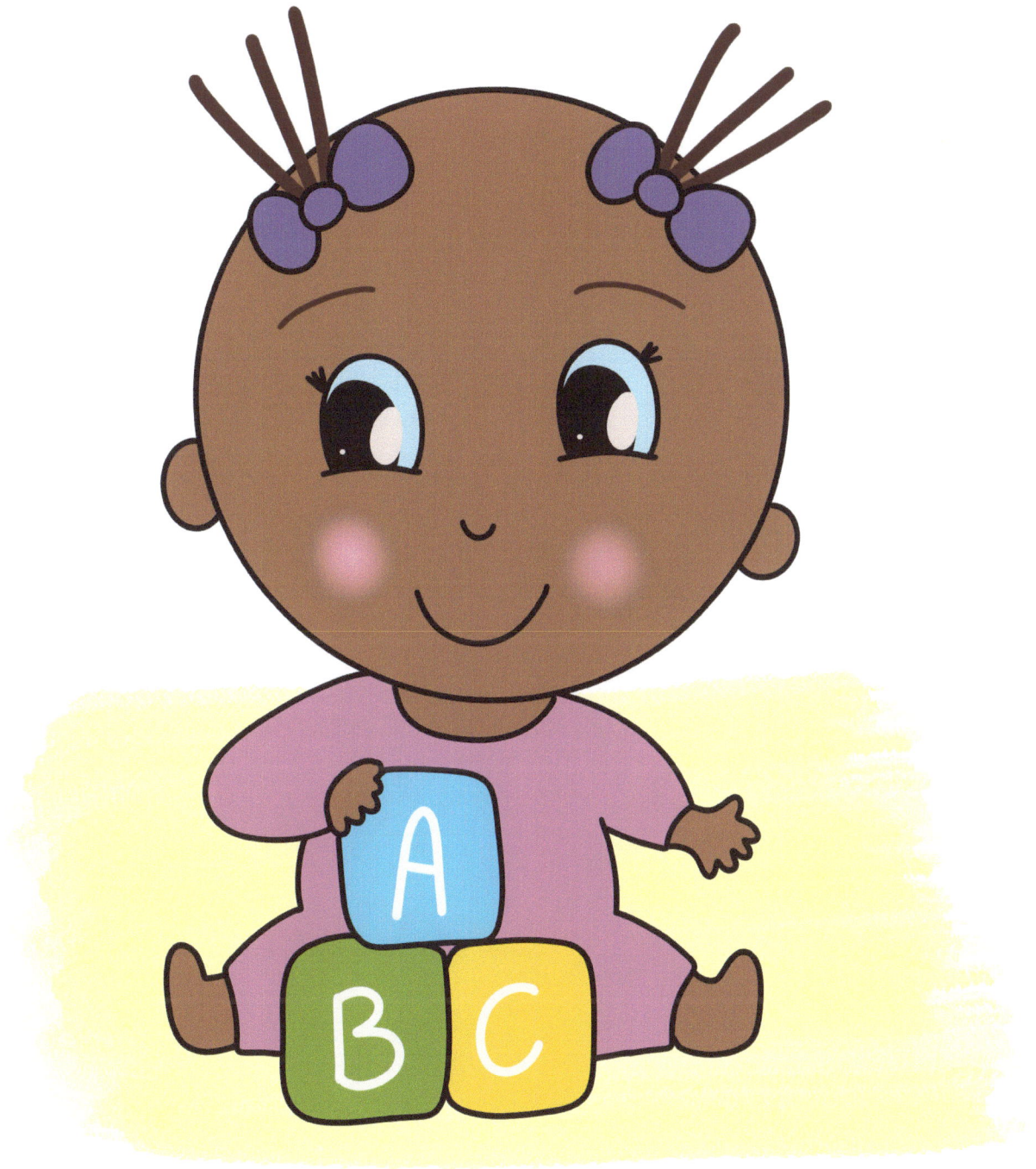

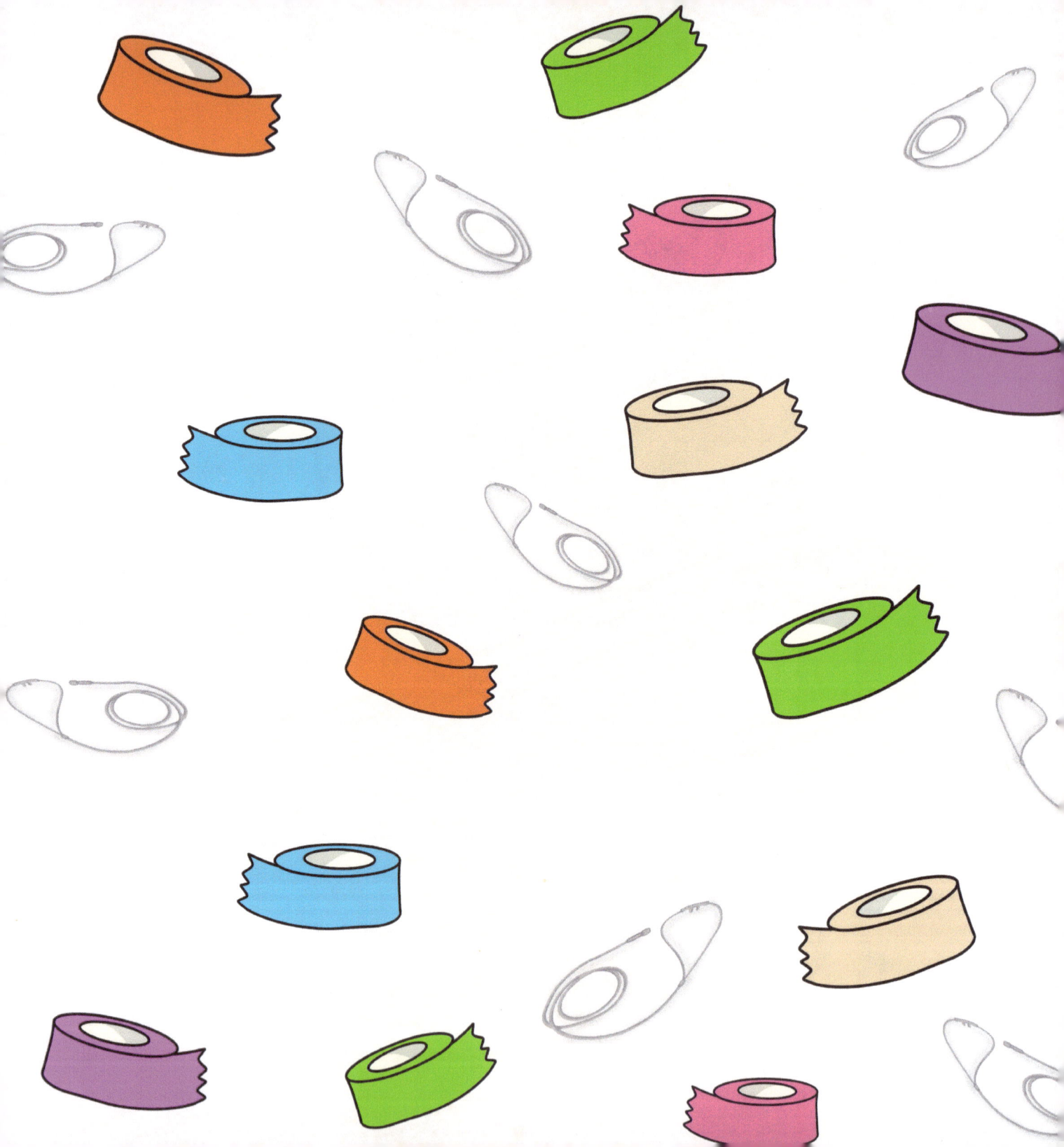

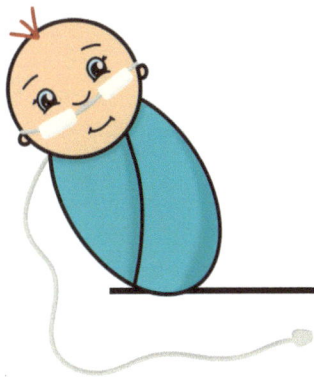

My Oxygen Baby

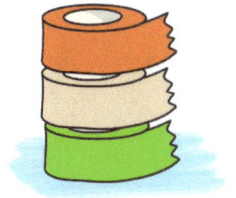

Name
_____

Diagnosis
_____

Date started oxygen
_____

Sleep Study & Home Oximeter Dates
_____
_____
_____

Date Stopped Oxygen!!
_____

How Many Days On Oxygen
_____

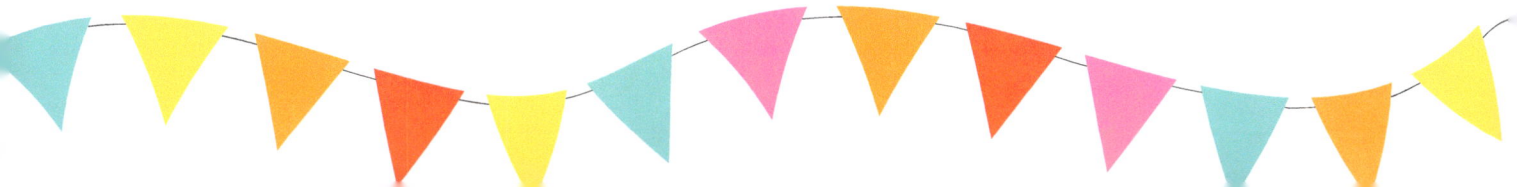

www.ingramcontent.com/pod-product-compliance
Lightning Source LLC
Chambersburg PA
CBHW061137030426

42334CB00003B/70